THE STUPID THINGS MY HUMAN DOES

TRUE STORIES FROM THE ER

D1366701

Narrated by: SEÑOR QUESO

(The cat on the cover)

DR. BARRIE SANDS

DEDICATION

By Señor Queso

This book is dedicated to the many different animals that have come through the emergency room who have taught me to love the life I live every moment, and to the brave and dedicated doctors, nurses, and support staff in the emergency room whose mission is to save lives, despite the stupid things you humans do.

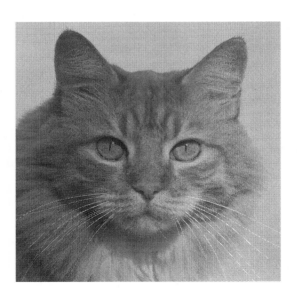

Table of Contents

WHY YOU SHOULD READ THE INTRODUCTION

Speaking for most, if not all cats; we tend to do things in our own time, and in our own way. As my friend the Cheshire Cat says with his ever mischievous smile; *"The proper order of things is often a mystery to me. You, too?"*

However...YOU are not a cat. It has come to my attention that some humans like to skip the introduction. The introduction of a book is like the first 15 minutes of a movie.... you don't want to miss it, especially this one. It is one of the few things that are actually written by the author, and it is a nice introduction to who I am. So, yes, it is important, impactful and in my feline opinion, not to be overlooked. Here is a quote from one of my favorite books. I think it says it all.

"Begin at the beginning," the King said, gravely, "and go on till you come to an end; then stop."
—Lewis Carroll, *Alice in Wonderland*

"Mistakes are a part of being human. Appreciate your mistakes for what they are: precious life lessons that can only be learned the hard way. Unless it is a fatal mistake, which, at least, others can learn from."

—Al Franken

INTRODUCTION

Life is filled with what we like to call "life lessons." These lessons are a part of a learning curve of how to navigate through the thralls of existence. At times, these lessons are tough and sometimes painful. The idea is to learn from them and try not to make the same mistake twice.

This sounds logical, but things in life don't always happen this way. There are a lot of factors involved in the events that take place. Some are within our control and some are not. So what now? What is the solution?

Sometimes the solution is finding wisdom in unexpected places. You don't need to burn your finger on a hot stove to know that it is hot. Your mother told you what would happen if you did. As children, we relied on and trusted that she was right and chose not to test out her "theory." In essence, we can learn from our own mistakes or we can learn from each other. I can tell you that learning from others is a lot less painful. It can also be fun.

We humans make mistakes, and yes, it would be great to learn from them, both our own and each other's. It is also important to maintain a sense of humor and to be able to laugh at ourselves in the process.

Let's face it, we already laugh at each other anyway, even if we don't want to admit it. It is part of human nature, so relax and gallantly saunter through the trials and tribulations in your life.

This book is about learning and laughing, and trying not to take ourselves so seriously. In the purview of serene lightheartedness, what better teacher is there than a cat? They have a knack for telling it like it is and not having an attachment to the emotional outcome.

At this point, you may be asking how can a cat write a book. Physically they can't. They lack opposable thumbs, and let's be honest, they don't even know how to type. However, even though they don't have the dexterity and required skills, they do have the ability to communicate and speak their minds. Anybody that lives with a cat would agree with me.

At this point, you may be wondering how I got caught up in this. How did this cat coerce me to write this book? For now, let's call it animal magnetism. Allow me, if you will, to tell you a little story.

THE STORY

It was a typical day in the hospital as I was sitting at my desk in the middle of the ER treatment room. I was ten hours into a fourteen-hour shift. All my senses were on high alert. I was listening to the background noises of dogs barking, doctors and nurses hustling around, and the grumbling sound of an empty and indignant stomach.

My eyes were glancing at the red blinking lights on the phone, clients and referring doctors waiting on hold to converse with me. At the same time, the intercom broadcasting from the front staff reception area informing us of critical animals coming to the back... STAT!

As I was trying to ignore the overhead pages beckoning me somewhere or another, I was encircled by a team of nurses holding up treatment sheets waiting patiently to ask me questions. Within that whirlwind-moment, being on the brink of a sensory systems overload, I suddenly remembered I had to go to the bathroom ... three hours ago and never went! I took a well-needed deep breath, announced to my staff that I will be in the bathroom for two minutes and walked away from the eternal chaos.

It was there in that ephemeral bubble of seclusion gathering my sanity when I realized that so many of the things that we see in the ER are *utterly preventable*, and at times ridiculously funny. In that moment, I started thinking about what I could do to change this madness.

Most people are unaware of what it is like to be an emergency room veterinarian. We are definitely in a unique and unclassified group of our own.

Being an ER veterinarian has its own special proclivities. We tend to bridge the gap between the studies of multispecies ethnography and the human epistemology of anthropomorphism. We not only treat our patients, the animals, but we also tend to the variety of needs of our clients—the people who cohabitate with the animals, care for, know, and love them.

Our patients, by conventional standards, are unable to tell us how they feel and what is bothering them. Therefore, we rely heavily on the use of our six senses. Yes six. We utilize the senses of touch, sight, smell, sound, taste, and the most important, the sixth sense—intuition. Mind you, we don't taste our patients, but it is nearly impossible not to "taste" the smells of hemorrhagic diarrhea from a puppy with Parvo viral enteritis. Yes, and in light of this, let's not forget the ever important seventh sense, our sense of humor.

Unlike human doctors, because our patients cannot speak, we rely on our ability to be good historians and get information from their owners. This is not as easy as one may think.

Most people who come to the ER are experiencing a multitude of negative and sometimes paralyzing emotions. The emotions of fear, anxiety, anger, sadness, and frustration activate the innate physiologic mechanisms of stress. It is very common that in those moments, other past events with similar emotional attachments are brought to the forefront of the consciousness. In those states, the neocortex or the frontal lobe "thinking" part of the brain automatically shuts down, and the "fight or flight" mechanisms take precedence.

When this happens, mental clarity, discernment, and inner calm basically go out the window. This tends to make my job that much more difficult, especially when I have an animal in a critical state and the only answers to my questions are, "I don't know."

Even though our patients do not speak, they do communicate. As such, I spend a great deal of time listening and talking to them. I learned to receive the information in a different way. This is where the sixth sense of intuition plays a key role.

As you may realize, as an emergency veterinarian, it is very important for us to be able to effectively communicate with our clients. As the primary guardians of our patients, clear communication with the "owners" is paramount. So how does one navigate through those situations? In order to circumvent the obvious stressors, it is important for us to maintain calm within the storm, to be a beacon of support and information, and to be an advocate for our patients. To do this, it is best to be in what is called a state of coherence.

Coherence is a physiological state of being when the heart, brain, and autonomic nervous system are in electrical, chemical, hormonal, and energetic alignment. The effect of this is a loving state of emotional neutrality, mental clarity, optimum physiologic function, and the recognition of the hearts' innate intelligence.

This allows me to be able to "listen" to the needs of my patients and clients more effectively. The techniques and teachings of heart-brain coherence are utilized by many emergency first responders such as navy SEALs, police task force, different governmental agencies, and many others. This subject is beyond the scope of this book, and if you would like more information, it can be found at the Institute of HeartMath web site. (https://www.heartmath.org/)

Day after day, week after week, year after year, I am always guaranteed to have a full and exciting day in the emergency room. Why? Because as we all know, metaphorically and realistically speaking, *shit* happens. It happens for many different reasons, and it happens EVERYWHERE. I do mean everywhere—on the floor, on the walls, on me, on the nursing staff ... everywhere. The word *crap* has taken on all sorts of new meanings.

This is the only job I know that the first words out of my mouth when I walk into work are, *"What is that smell?"* And yes, I love my job! Please forgive my mephitic digression.

Now to be serious, being slightly frustrated by the plethora of things that I see and treat gave me the idea to write a book about what goes on in the ER. But it wasn't until I met Señor Queso, the cat on the cover of this book, that the thought to write a book really started to feel like a necessity. I guess he inspired me, not because he came to our hospital due to something "stupid that a human did," but because HE had something he wanted to say; I just had to help him say it.

How did we meet? Well, I'll leave those details up to him to tell, but for me, our true relationship started when I walked into the ER phone room and found him there. The phone room is a quiet place where the doctors can get away to think, write records, make phone calls, and yet still be able to see what is going on in the ICU, triage area. One day, I walked into the phone room to find this adorably handsome orange cat happily eating MY blueberry muffin.

Señor Queso, nonchalantly looked up at me, offered me a fleeting glance of what I can only describe as blithe indifference, and went back to eating my muffin. I commandeered what was left of the muffin and inquired to the staff as to how he got in there.

They proceeded to explain that they wanted to give him an opportunity to stretch, move about, and get a little exercise. They said they felt sorry for him "being cooped up" in his cage, and proclaimed that it was, in actuality, all his idea. I could already see that this cat had a substantive, almost hypnotic influence over people. As for me, I can honestly say, it was in that moment I knew there was something special between us. Even though I was upset about my muffin, it was hard to be upset with him.

Queso (as we call him), stayed with us in the hospital for a while. During the time he was there, he witnessed hundreds of different incidents and wanted to convey the stories from his perspective. As it turned out, he had conversations with many of the patients. My purpose and function for the undertaking of writing this book was to comply and be of assistance. As you may know, if you live with a cat, they can be very persuasive and, let's not forget, they lack the ability to type.

To be forewarned, Queso is a devilishly irresistible cat. He is probably the most personable cat that I have ever met. He can also be a little sassy, as you will find out, but it is all part of his charm. Keep in mind that I am only the messenger. He has some great stories and pearls of wisdom. Like me, I know that you will find him charismatic and extremely funny. It's ok if you fall in love with him; I'll understand—some things are very easy to do.

"A cat has absolute emotional honesty: human beings, for one reason, or another, may hide their feelings, but a cat does not."

—Ernest Hemingway

WHERE IT ALL BEGAN: TELLING IT LIKE IT IS

Offended by the title? Well, this book is long overdue. Allow me to introduce myself.

I am a cat, but not just any cat. My name is Señor Queso. That's right—Mr. Cheese. I also go by the name King Queso Meso McFuzzy Butt. (I'll get to that story later.)

My human, to put it mildly, is awesome! She is one of those humans that is almost as smart as cats. Sometimes she is even smarter, *if* you can believe that is possible. You see, my human is an animal doctor. They call themselves veterinarians. (It's ok; it took me awhile to get THAT name right too). They hang out in a place called a "Specialty Hospital." Apparently she is part of an elite team of veterinarians. They call themselves Emergency Critical Care Doctors. That's right; they are the top-notch, the brave, the cleaner uppers, and fixers of stupidity. How do I know? Well, that's the story isn't it? I spent time in this place and I've seen some crazy cat shit go down, and these humans do stuff that I never thought possible. Let me start with my personal story of how I got caught up in all of this.

FINDING MY WAY TO THE HOSPITAL

Ok, did I mention that I live in San Diego? Great place to grow up. As a young stud, I spent most of my time outside. Running through the grass, climbing trees, jumping on rooftops, and catching birds (don't judge me!). I am quite a hunter and love to get in touch with my inner tiger. I am wise to the ways of the suburban jungle.

Then one sunny day, I was outside doing my usual thing, running around chasing butterflies, when I got attacked by a patch of these tall, spikey sticky pokey plant things. Stopped me dead in my tracks! They were all over me. It hurt, and every time I tried to move it felt like I was getting smothered by an army of puffer fish. I don't know how many there were attacking; it felt like hundreds, no thousands! It didn't matter—until I noticed, *The One*, the one that would change my life forever. The One, that was in a place where the sun does not shine. I just laid there sad and pathetic, unable to go any further... waiting for somebody to come.

And then I saw her... my human. (This is not the human that I am with now; we are getting to that). I let out some cries of help and she came running.

She was sweet, always good to me, let me do want I wanted, fed me ... yeah she was nice. She came over to me and stared at me for a little while. I felt like an exposed porcupine. (In hindsight, I think she was trying to figure out just what to do with me.) "Hurry up!" I said, "Quit staring and do something ... Please!"

She picked me up, wrapped me in a soft towel, and drove me to this building. Yes, the Specialty Hospital, where I met *HER*... my NEW human. Why new human? Well, as you say, the plot thickens.

This doctor started to examine me, and although I was covered with these plants that she called Foxtails, it was after she noticed *The One* that the look on her face changed and she called out for some *pain medication*. This was supposed to make me feel better and it did! I felt a small pinch-like poke and then, Aaaahhh ... Yes! My prayers were answered.

There was a lot of fussing over me and most things were a little hazy. I don't know just how long I was in that state, but the next thing I knew I woke up with a Pagina! A Pagina? What's that you say? Leaving out the gory details, it is basically making a male body part into a female body part.

How did this happen, you ask? Well, as I was waking up I overheard the nurses and doctors discussing my unique situation. They said that a foxtail was stuck in my urethra—yes that was *The One!* Now you understand.

Well, as it happens, there was a significant amount of damage to my urethra and they needed to surgically remove it and create a new opening; hence my Pagina. Please, no need for your sympathy; it worked out great! Haven't had a problem since, and it allowed me to get in touch with my "Sacred Feminine Feline" (did I say that out loud?).

Anyway, as it turned out, I traded my surgery for the noble service of Blood Donorship. (I'll get to those details later). You see, my old human wasn't able to pay for my care so I guess, because I was so handsome, they offered to do the necessary surgery in exchange for my giving back to the feline community. The only caveat was that my old owner would have to give me up and I would get a new home after my donorship was over. You can say it was "blood money."

So here it was, my new home. Home sweet home. I was in a cage. Imagine ME in a cage. The Stealthy Hunter, the Roamer of Hills, the Chaser of Butterflies, the Free in the Freedom. Yes, this was to be my new life, for now.

It was actually not as bad as I thought it would be. I had a warm soft bed, a clean bathroom, plenty of food, and nurses that would constantly love on me (again, because I was so irresistibly handsome). Oh, and let me not forget to mention the incredible amount of endless entertainment.

The emergency room is a busy place. I soon found out that I was not alone. There were a few other cats in this elite special ops program. They had a nice set up where they would hang out and wait until they were needed.

They lived in a larger room with a nice view of the outside world and got to hang out in these things they called cat trees. Not like the ones I was used to, but it was ok. The next few months, however, I was in a Quarantine Phase—I guess to make sure my blood was pristine for the ones that may need it.

During this time, I had the opportunity to check out the establishment and see what goes on. Oh the stories I could tell you! Wait ... Right. That's what I'm doing here.

There are so many stories, hard to decide on which ones. The emergency room was opened 24/7/365. That means ALL THE TIME! It was a very busy place. Some days and times were busier than others, but for the majority of the time, all the beds were being used and at times it was standing room only. Yep. There is NO shortage of stories. I am now going to share some of these stories with you.

E.R., the final frontier.

These are the stories of the Emergency Critical Care Hospital. My four month mission: To explore strange new phenomena, to seek out new experiences and new occurrences, to boldly go where no cat has gone before... Da da dana na na na...

Ok, now be prepared. Some of these stories are very funny and some are very sad, even tragic. But let me just say, as an Ambassador of Animals, we understand that you are ONLY HUMAN, and humans make mistakes and do silly, crazy, and sometimes just down right stupid things. Now don't feel SO bad about yourselves. Come on. Admit it. You are always calling each other stupid anyway. We want you to know that we forgive you and love you regardless.

In general, dogs are more forgiving than us cats. It is known that dogs are beacons of unconditional love and want to be of service, and as truth be told, we cats are here to teach you a thing or two. As such, I have added a moral at the end of these stories, as part of a take home message, in hopes that it may limit the stupid things you humans do.

These are true stories. The names have been changed to "protect the innocent."

"Only two things are infinite, the universe and human stupidity, and I'm not sure about the former."

—Albert Einstein

CRUSTY

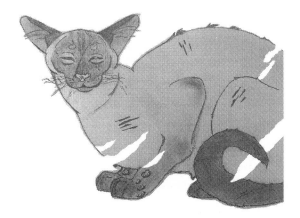

It was a busy Saturday morning when a cat was rushed back to the treatment area. (In the ER it seemed like mostly everything got "rushed" back to the treatment area.) I guess it was because they needed immediate attention, and let me say, these doctors are fast.

So, this cat was rushed back in a cardboard box. When they opened the box, there was a cute Siamese who I called Crusty. Her face looked as if it was burnt. Her whiskers were singed, her nose and lips were red and puffy, her eyes were closed, and her head was bright red. When they took her out of the box, you could see that all her paws were red and swollen and some parts even had blisters. Ouch, that looked painful. She did not seem very happy. The doctor took a good look at her. They call it an examination. I then heard one of the doctors request pain medication.

"Oh yeah!" I thought. She will feel a lot better soon. The doctor gave her the injection and placed her on a soft blanket while she went to speak with the humans. This gave me a chance to talk to her.

"Hi Crusty," I said. "What happened to you?"

She said that her name wasn't Crusty, but she didn't mind me calling her that. She said that she went into this opening that had a door and took a nap on some clothes and the next thing she knew, she was spinning, flopping, and being banged around. The door was closed, and it was getting very hot inside. She wasn't sure how long she was in there, but she said her humans came just in time. She thought she was going to pass out.

Just then, the doctor came back with the scoop (that means story) and said that the "owners," as they are called, were lying in bed and kept hearing this banging noise coming from the garage. The female asked the male if he had put his sneakers in the dryer.

He thought about it and said, "No." Then moments later they looked at each other and yelled, *"THE CAT!"* then immediately ran into the garage and opened the dryer to find Miss Crusty huffing and puffing.

Miss Crusty ended up staying in the hospital for a couple of days as they treated her burns and gave her medication for the pain and antibiotics to help fight infections. The doctors told the owners how to take care of her when they got home and that it would take a little while until she was good as new, but she should make a full recovery. I wished her well and off she went.

Moral of the Story:

Cats are not dryer safe! In the future, keep the dryer doors closed and before you do, always check to see that nobody is in there taking a nap. As you may not know, we cats are very curious and love to nap on clothes.

ALI

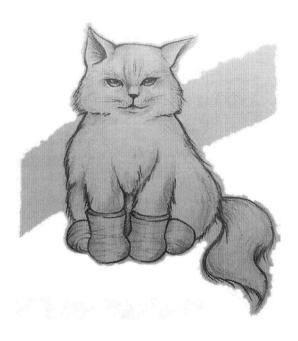

It was a regular busy day in the ER when this silvery white long-haired cat came in. He looked very clean, and he smelled good. He was standing there on the treatment table constantly shaking each one of his paws, one after the other. He seemed very upset. Upon each paw, he was wearing these greyish, silver booties that looked like boxing gloves. He would take a swing at anybody that tried to get close to him.

I said, "Hey Ali! Nice boxing gloves."

He looked at me, hissed, and said, "These are NOT boxing gloves."

Yup. He was very mad! He seemed like a pretty wild dude that didn't like to take anything from anybody.

The doctor went to talk to his owner and find out what had happened. She came back laughing to herself and shaking her head. "What's up?" I said.

She started to explain to her nurses what she needed to do to help Ali. It turns out that Mr. Ali needed a bath, and because of his fine and cooperative disposition (NOT!), his owners, in trying to prevent getting mauled by Mr. Ali before his bath, decided that it was a good idea to wrap a bunch of duct tape around each foot. Hence, the boxing gloves.

Well, what they didn't take into consideration was that it was going to be impossible to get the duct tape off! And so ... here he was.

Soon Mr. Ali got some of that magic pain medication and finally relaxed. The doctors and nurses worked on taking off his gloves for a little while, and after some gentle cutting and soaking and use of some magic anti-sticky stuff, they were able to free his feet. They even gave him a nail trim. He seemed happier afterwards, but still pretty grumpy.

They sent him home with some stuff to soak his feet in for a day or so to help with the irritation. "Good luck with that!" I said to Ali. "At least you smell good!"

He hissed back at me as he went out the door. Charming fellow!

Moral of the Story:

The use of duct tape should be reserved for automotive and housing projects. Not CATS! Or Snakes (but that's another story).

SHERLOCK

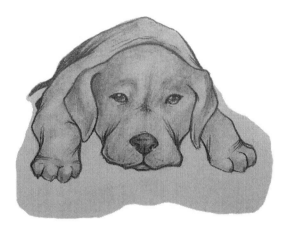

This is a little bit of a longer story, but it is a goody. You'll understand his name later.

Sherlock was a big, black Labrador Retriever. I am not much of a dog lover, but I have to say, he was pretty cute. He came into the ER walking, but very slowly; his head and tail were down. I don't know about you, but when a Labrador doesn't move his tail, something is really wrong. I mean these guys seem to live for the use of that tail. It is a direct extension of their brain (if you can call it that).

So I ask him, "Hey Chum, why so glum?"

He says his belly hurts and even though he still wants to eat (that's a Lab for you), he vomits everything right back up. He hasn't kept anything down for days. "That's terrible," I exclaimed. "But don't worry – you came to the right place. These humans here are really helpful".

The doctor came over to look at him and he moaned when they touched his belly. They gave him a good once over and decided that he needed to stay in the hospital, have some tests run, and get him started on feeling better.

The doctor spoke to the owner; she was a pretty lady. She was very sad and wasn't much help. She did say that he had a habit of eating things that he shouldn't, but that he never seemed to have a problem before. She came by his bedside, gave him a kiss and a hug, and told him she would see him later. That was nice; he really seemed to like that.

So... the doctors put an IV catheter in him (that is an Intravenous – for all you non-medical types), attached a bag of liquid (they call it fluids), and started to give it to him. That seemed to make him feel more perky. His tail started to wag. "Way to go Sherlock!" I said.

Next, they took him all over the hospital. He got to ride on this thing called a gurney. He went into Radiology to get X-rays, and then to a place called The Ultrasound Room, where he got an ultrasound of his abdomen, and then he came back to his bed. He looked like he was having fun.

The doctors were all huddled together talking about him and then decided that he needed surgery. He looked a little worried. "I had surgery," I told Sherlock. "It was a piece of cake. They give you this 'pain medication' and then you wake up with a Pagina—it's all good!"

Ha! You should have seen his face when I told him that! Dogs ... they are so gullible.

"No seriously!" I told him. "This surgery thing happens a lot and everyone is different. These doctors do a really great job. They will fix you right up."

SO fast forward ... He is waking up from his procedure, sleeping like a baby, drool and all, and the doctors are talking to the owner lady.

They are telling her that her dog was going to be fine and that they found a pair of panties stuck in his intestines. They even showed them to her; they were a little yucked up from living inside the dog for a few days, but they looked like a lacey red thong. The owner looked at the panties and her face immediately changed. She looked mad! And then she exclaimed, "These are not my underwear; I don't wear red lace thongs!"

Way to go Sherlock!

Well, as it turned out, Mr. Sherlock broke the case of the "Cheating Husband" and after the brake up, proceeded to live with the nice lady who brought him in.

Moral of the Story:

If you are going to cheat on your significant other then don't have a Labrador. Or better yet, don't wear underwear.

THE ELEPHANT IN THE ROOM

OK, I need to get this off my chest and address the elephant in the treatment room. Now, for all you dog lovers out there, we need to discuss this thing they call the Bulldog. What makes me an expert on Bulldogs? Nothing, I am just a cat doin' time and it seems that these guys are in here an awful lot. It's like a weekly convention. They come in for all sorts of stuff. I hate to say it, but I think a lot of it has to do with their faces! As cute as it may seem, it is quite inefficient. It's all squished up and the nose holes are way too small. Perhaps that is why they make such a weird sound (like a lawn mower in heat), even when they are just standing still.

Let me tell you about Blue.

BLUE

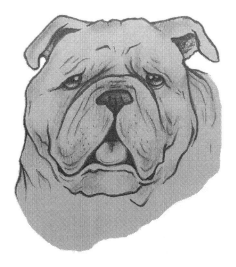

Right. So … One hot day in July, in comes Blue, why Blue? Because that was the color of his tongue when I met him. Even I know that blue tongues are never ok. He didn't look so good. He was on one of those gurneys, lying there trying to breathe. He looked hot and calorically challenged. (That's politically correct isn't it?). They took a thermometer and put it in his rear end (they call it a rectum), and then everything became very busy after that! There were lots of doctors and nurses doing all sorts of things.

Someone said his temperature was 109.7 degrees! Wow, I didn't even think that was possible. The doctors and nurses spent the next few minutes cooling him down; and doing all sorts of other stuff. They even had to place a tube down his throat. I think it was to help him breathe, because his tongue became pink after that. They worked fast. I was pretty impressed with these humans.

When it seemed like things were under control and Blue was starting to look better, the doctor left to go talk to the owner.

As it turns out, Blue and his owner were on a "run" in the park, and Blue just collapsed. Hmmm, Ok, let me get this straight. This guy and his smushed faced, no nose hole, overweight Bulldog were out on a "RUN" in the park in the middle of July. Now I ask you ... What part of THAT seemed like a good idea?

Well as it turned out, Mr. Blue was in pretty bad shape for a few days. He suffered from a bad case of Heatstroke. I didn't think he was going to make it out of the hospital. But he did. He slowly recovered and went home to run another day. Maybe this time ... in the winter.

> **Moral of the Story:**
>
> **If you have a Bulldog that likes to run, maybe think about going to a movie instead.**

—*~*~*—

Since we are on the topic of Bulldogs ... Here's another story.

MR. SEXY

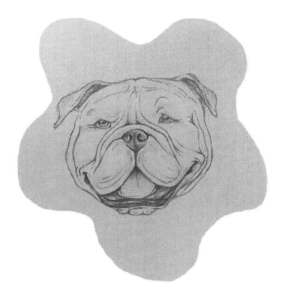

Yes, Mr. Sexy is his REAL name. I know what I said before, but I just couldn't change it because well, he actually was ... kinda Sexy in his own way, and perhaps not so innocent, but who am I to say. His story is simple—Mr. Sexy spent his days not doing too much, which is completely appropriate for a Bulldog. He came into the ER during the summer. Even though he too came in on a gurney (much like Blue), he didn't seem so bad.

He was sitting up looking around. Sort of like Jabba the Hutt mated with an Ottoman. As he rolled by I said, "Hey Mr. Sexy, what brings you in here?"

He looked at me with this rather cute but dumb look on his face and said, and I am not joking, "I don't know, I was just sittin' on my porch just hangin' out, doin' my thing and started to feel a little dizzy and couldn't walk so well. It's very hot outside today ... ya know?"

I just nodded and smiled. Really, what else can one say after something like that?

So after the usual once over, the good doctors thought he was mildly overheated but otherwise seemed ok. They ended up giving him a couple of cold packs, recommended to hold off on the Twinkies, and talked to the owners about doing some kind of surgery and sent him home.

Moral of the Story:

Feeling sexy is one thing but being "hot" has a whole new meaning if you are overweight, and respiratorily (I know that is not a real word but I like it, and I'm a cat so I can do what I want), challenged.

INFORMATION INTERLUDE

Unlike you humans, we do not "sweat." It is quite unbecoming of a cat. We get rid of heat and regulate our body temperature by this glamorous thing we do when we open our mouths and stick out our tongues. It is called panting! Air exchange via the mouth and nose is a very important part of us keeping cool. We cats don't pant *as much* as dogs; we are usually pretty good at "chillin'" if you know what I mean.

Keep in mind that you do not need to have a smushed face to become overheated. This happens in many other kinds of dogs. It usually involves a hot day, a hike, a ball, a Frisbee, or some other hypnotic fetching device and an endless desire to play. The effects of "heat stroke," as the doctors call it, can be deadly. So please, take it from a cat and try to keep cool.

Ok, I am sure you are all wondering about the "surgery" that they talk about for these guys. Even though this is not what I intended to share with you, it may be helpful in keeping these dogs out of the ER and taking up so much space.

Listen carefully, like I said, I am not an expert, but I do hear a lot of talking. Smushed face dogs (not just Bulldogs because there are many other kinds out there) have a condition they call "Brachycephalic Airway

Syndrome," which translates into "Smushed face, can't breathe, all messed up, need's help." That's my own interpretation. If you happen to be one of those humans that likes to be around these dogs then I advise you to speak to your own veterinarian about the details.

Oh by the way ... here is another tid bit. Now there are always exceptions to the rule, but most Bulldogs are not good swimmers! They have a tendency to want to sink like rocks. There is a saying "sink or swim, heads or tails?" Well, where Bulldogs are concerned, it's "Sink ... bottom's up!" If you do want your Bulldog to be a water baby then you may want to invest in a good floatation device.

Ok enough about these guys. Let's talk about another species. After all, the ER is a non-discriminatory place—all sorts of critters come in. They see birds, rabbits, turtles, ferrets, guinea pigs (or G.pigs as they are referred to), and all kinds of reptiles—iguanas, chameleons, and snakes. Heck, I once saw an Emu waltz in with his tail feathers all messed up. He ended up getting attacked by the dog in the house and got his butt all bit up. I think the dog thought he was helping out for the Thanksgiving holiday. See, we cats are not the only ones that like to hunt for our dinner.

Ok, here is a story about a snake.

NIBBLES

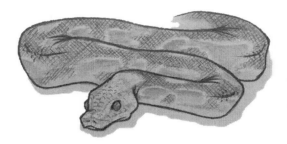

Nibbles was a really long Ball Python. I have to tell you that I do not like snakes. I had a few run ins with them in the good ol' days, and it never ended well for the snake. But when he came in, I actually felt a little sorry for the chap.

Allow me to digress for a moment. In the ER, not everybody gets rushed to the back; some sit up front and wait to be seen. It depends upon how "critical" you are. It is usually NEVER GOOD when you are the first one seen in the ER! Please try to remember that when you are waiting PATIENTLY for hours to be seen!

Anyway, the charts have these stickers on them with information and what they call a "presenting complaint." That's what the human owner writes down.

So, Nibbles sticker said *Presenting Complaint: "Attacked by Dinner."*

Pretty funny huh? Well not so much for poor Nibbles. So he comes back in a glass box, he's just lying there; he had these small wounds all over him. I say to him as he came by, holding back my Ninja moves, "Hey Nibbles! What's eating you?"

He looked at me a little embarrassed and said one word, "Dinner."

"How did that happen?" I asked with tender Cat Curiosity. He explained that it was time for his weekly meal, and from out of nowhere, like on a stealth mission, dropped into his cage a rather large robust mouse. This "Mighty Mouse" proceeded to open up a "Can of Whoop Ass," and Nibbles became the meal. Like I said, poor Nibbles, trapped in a small space with an assassin mouse. Well lucky for him, the good doctors knew just how to help.

They cleaned his wounds, gave him the magic pain medication and a shot of an antibiotic. He was very cooperative and appreciative. They sent him home with some stuff to help keep the wounds clean. I'm pretty sure he will make a full recovery. He seemed like a pretty cool dude. Maybe I need to reconsider my feelings about snakes.

Moral of the Story:

One should EAT dinner, not get eaten BY dinner. And in my personal opinion, dinner is not dinner until is it served on a plate accompanied by a glass of warm milk.

Since we are on the topic of snakes, here's another story.

HOUDINI

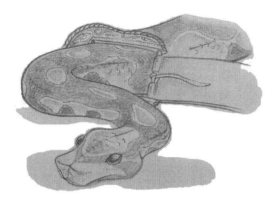

Ok so here comes another Python (I guess they are popular with the humans). Houdini was ... STUCK! Ha ha. This may not be as much as what a Stupid Human Does as it is what a stupid snake did.

Houdini's owner looked like a cowboy, biker dude—you know the type. Driving around on those things with two wheels that make lots of noise? I believe they call it a motorcycle. He had long hair, pictures all over his skin, and was wearing a leather vest, jeans, boots, and a belt with a BIG buckle. He seemed really chill.

I could picture myself riding tandem with the wind blowing through my whiskers. If it wasn't for the snake, I might have been tempted to ask him to break me out of here.

Anyway—back to the snake. So here was poor Houdini, stuck! I asked him. "How did you get yourself into this mess? It looks like it hurts!"

He said it did. He was out and about slithering around when he decided to go through this really cool looking square thing. He got about halfway through when he got stuck. He said he's been stuck for a while as his owner and friends were trying to push and pull him out. Nothing was working and he was becoming very swollen. He was stuck in one of his owner's really cool looking belt buckles.

The doctor came over to examine him and decided that they needed to cut him loose. They gave him some of that great pain medication and when he was relaxed, they got out these rather large looking bolt cutters and cut the buckle, while protecting the snake from any further harm. They were very successful! The area of his body that was stuck was red, swollen, and irritated, but the doctors thought he would be back to normal in a couple of days.

Houdini was very grateful and as he left he said to me, "You know I probably could have made it if it wasn't for the rat I ate shorty before that."

I said, "Yep those crazy rodents, causing all sorts of trouble ... you may want to consider becoming a vegetarian."

He stuck out his funny looking tongue and slithered away. I think that was him trying to laugh.

Moral of the Story:

Never look a gift buckle in the mouth ... at least not until you have digested your dinner. There is a saying that "curiosity killed the cat." Well, at least we don't get stuck in belt buckles.

FLASHBACK

Remember a little while ago when I was talking about duct tape and I mentioned an incident with a snake? Well, long story short, there was a snake that came in because the kids at home wanted to experiment with the snake and the duct tape. They proceeded to duct tape the snake's mouth open. I know what you're thinking— you'd have to see it to believe it. Use your imagination.

The poor snake was very unhappy, not to mention how angry the parents were. Have no fear; in the end it all worked out ok for the snake, but I don't think I can say the same about the kids.

Moral of that Story:

When the parents are away, the kids will play ... or get into trouble. It might be best to keep an eye or two on those small humans.

GALILEO

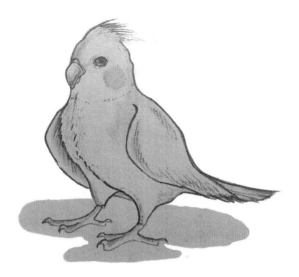

Even though I like to chase birds (really, it is just anything that flies; it allows me to practice my aerial skills), I do feel badly for them when they come into the ER. Here is a story about a brave bird named Galileo.

Galileo was a Cockatiel. He was a smallish bird. He was grey and white and had a yellow head with orange cheeks. He came back in a cage. He did not look good at all. He was sitting at the bottom of the cage with his head down and was all puffed up. He didn't even want to talk me. The doctor quickly examined him and placed him inside an oxygen cage. She looked very concerned. I had a bad feeling about this one. The doctor went to go talk to the owner to find out more about the situation.

She came back with a sad look on her face and checked on Galileo. He looked even worse. She didn't look surprised. The sad story is that Galileo was in the kitchen, whistling and dancing around earlier that day, and then proceeded to get very weak and puffy.

As it turns out, the owner was cooking—cause that's what you tend to do in kitchens—and she happens to cook on these pots and pans that are "non-stick" coated with a chemical called Teflon. Ok—here's where I sound really smart. Teflon when heated emits these odorless, colorless toxic fumes called Polytetrafluoroethylene (PTFE) for short.

Birds are very sensitive to these fumes and other kinds of gaseous chemicals. It is considered a Killer of Birds. Even though humans are not that sensitive, I have heard that it is toxic to humans as well. You might want to look into that.

Sadly, despite the doctors efforts, little Galileo did not make it, and the owner took him home for a proper birdy burial.

There is an old saying, "A canary in a coal mine." It is not just a song written by this 80's rock band called The Police. It is a true story that tells of the use of canaries as a sentinel species for coal miners in the early 1900's. Due to the birds' sensitive and unique respiratory system, they can detect odorless gasses by well ... DYING, and therefore warned the miners of these toxic gases. Thankfully this detection system stopped in the late 1980s.

SO the Moral of this Story:

Don't treat your bird as a "canary in a coal mine" and look into investing in much better cookware, because the life you save could be your own.

MARTY

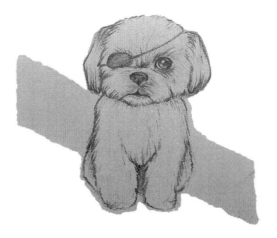

There are, on occasion, those situations that you don't want to look at but can't seem to take your eye off of. Sometimes the stuff that we see is kinda' gross. Everybody has a different threshold for a "gross out" factor. For some, it's eyeballs; but I think they are weirdly interesting.

We heard the overhead page, "Tech to the front STAT," and a few moments later a nurse came rushing back carrying a small dog wrapped in a blanket. Behold Marty.

Marty is a bug eyed Shih Tzu. For those who don't know, a Shih Tzu has a small face with eyes that are big and bulgy. Marty was wrapped in the blanket with his head exposed and his eyeball popped out of his head! Yep, definitely yucky but cool, in a creepy sort of way.

I didn't get a chance to talk to him before the doctors took him away to examine. They looked him over to see if he was in shock, gave him some pain medications, and tried to assess if they could save the eye and have him be able to see again. After they did all that, they concluded that the trauma was only to his face, and he was not in a state of shock, (although I think some of the surrounding humans were). The doctor then went into a room to talk to the owner humans.

This gave me a chance to talk to poor Marty. I asked him how his eye fell out of his head. As he looked up at me, I could see his weird eye still trying to move around to find me. Cool and again…slightly creepy. He told me that it all happened very fast; everything was a little blurry. Ha!

He recalled that he and his human family were very excited to go for a drive in the car. He wasn't sure where they were going, but it was going to be a lot of fun. Everybody was busy hustling about getting into the car.

Marty said because he was short he had to take a running start to get into the back seat, and right after he jumped, in midair, he felt his head get smashed. He wasn't sure what happened after that, but he said his head hurt and he couldn't see well, and he ended up in the hospital. He said he did feel a little better after he got some of the pain medication.

When the doctor came back from the room, she said that the owner didn't see him jumping into the car and slammed the car door on his head. Ouch! The doctor also said that based upon her assessment and because they rushed him in right after the incident happened, she thinks she can save the eye and he should be able to see. That was really good news.

The doctor and staff did not waste any time in preparing for and performing his procedure. I overheard something about worrying about the optic nerve being stretched for too long. Anyway, they put him under anesthesia, and with impressive technical skill, they basically pushed his eyeball back into the socket and then sutured his eyelids together to make sure the eye would not fall out again. They said that this was only temporary until the eye healed and the swelling went away.

Marty was able to go home after he woke up from this procedure. He left with some of those good pain medications, eye drops, and a party hat, or the cone of shame, as I like to call it.

> **Moral of the Story:**
>
> **A dog is part of the family, not a squeeze toy; and remember, they say "it is all fun and games, until somebody loses an eye," or in Marty's case, pops one out.**

DOWN RIGHT HILARIOUS

Ok, now sometimes something walks in that is just down right hilarious and not only because of the situation, but because of what the doctors and nurses say. Mind you, I am not here to make anybody feel bad— just to share some funny stuff. Do you know how funny something needs to be to get a cat to laugh?

AGNUS

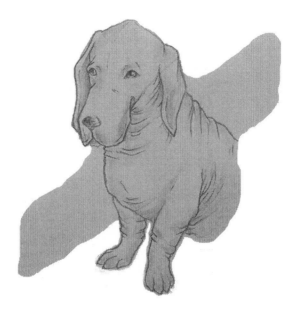

So, in walks this old female dog named Agnus. The owner said she was having a problem with something "down there" as she gestured to her lower "private" body parts. Agnus was yellowish brown with a short coat and looked like a Labrador mixed with a Basset hound. She was already kinda funny looking. She had a head like a Labrador and legs like a Basset Hound and a body that was the mix of the two.

She was standing in the treatment area wagging her tail, waiting to be examined when Doctor A walked by and said "Woa! What is that!?" referring to her rear end.

Doctor B said, "THAT is a VULVA."

Doctor C walked over and said, "That is the BIGGEST vulva I have ever seen!"

Doctor B said, "Yes that is why she is here."

Nurse A asked, "How does a vulva get like that?"

Doctor C said, "It looks old and over used."

Doctor A asked, "What are you going to do about that vulva?"

Doctor B said, "I don't know if there is anything you CAN do about that vulva, it may just be an old, flabby vulva."

Just then Agnus looked at me and asked, "Why are they all talking about my vulva? What's wrong with it? It seems fine to me."

I couldn't help but just stare at her laughing (on the inside—of course).

Poor Agnus. I don't think her vulva got that much attention in a long time, or perhaps maybe that was part of the problem. You know dogs and their love of "Genital Salutations!"

As it turned out, Miss Agnus had a few litters in her lifetime and her owner was allowing Agnus to get into situations that she may have been just too old for. She was just experiencing a little temporary irritation "down there."

The doctor sent her home with an antiseptic wash for a few days and recommended that Agnus not have any more "playdates," if you know what I mean.

Moral of the Story:

No matter how many times I think about this story ... it still makes me laugh and laughter is always the best medicine; and even though there are oldies but goodies, there comes a time in one's life when you need to put the old horse out to pasture.

Sorry Agnus.

TWITCH

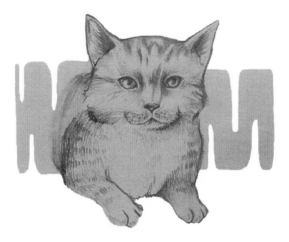

Ok, I'm going to get a little serious here. Some of these stories are "no harm no foul," but some of the things that you humans do can have dire consequences.

So, in comes this cat … she was a cute grey and white Tabby. I called her Twitch. She was rushed to the back, wrapped in a towel. She was just lying there staring at something. She looked like she might have been dead, except if you looked closely she was still breathing and every once in a while her body would twitch.

The doctor rushed over to her and within moments was requesting permission with the lady on the phone to do all sorts of things. I think she was talking to someone up front, maybe the receptionist, and they were talking to the owner. The nurses got busy getting blood work and placing the IV catheter. When they got results of her blood sugar ... the machine said *"LO."* That means really LOW.

I heard the doctor say that this cat was very "hypo-glycemic" (that means low blood sugar). They gave her some liquid sugar into her IV catheter. After that, she became less twitchy, and as she was started on some other treatments, the doctor went to talk to the owner.

Ok, so they found out that the cat has a condition called Diabetes and she gets Insulin shots every day to help her. Now let me take a moment to explain this, because this is important. There are A LOT of cats out there that have this condition—I know because they come in to the ER. Some are first timers that are just figured out, or *diagnosed,* as they say in doctor land, and others are here for complications—like Twitch.

It seems to me that you humans do not understand what Diabetes is all about. So in the name of "Self-Species Preservation," I will try to educate you a little. Once again, I am not an expert, but I have seen this far too many times and I think the doctors get tired of talking about it.

Diabetes is a *very complicated* process, and involves very complex metabolic reactions. Even I don't understand all of it, and I am pretty smart. So here's the simplified "info on the down low."

Diabetes = High blood glucose

Glucose is a form of sugar that the body likes to use for fuel and energy; it comes from the food we eat. (It's not the same form of sugar that is in Mr. Sexy's Twinkies).

Why is the glucose in the blood high?

The body is not able to make, or efficiently use, this protein called insulin. (Like I said it's complicated, but don't worry).

Why does that matter?
The job of insulin is to help put glucose into cells.

Who cares?
Simple answer ... You Do!

The cells in the body NEED glucose to live, and if it is hanging around in the blood stream then the cells are STARVING. And when you starve—YOU DIE! Get it?

So how do you get the glucose from the blood stream to go into the cells? Easy Peasy Lemon Squeezy!

You give insulin injections! Ok, hopefully some of you are starting to get a grasp on the situation.

So back to my poor feline friend Twitch ... Even though the doctor gave her glucose injections, her blood glucose was better but still lower than it should be.

She looked a little more lively, but not really. I could tell that this fix was going to take some time.

So what happened to her? I just told you that when you have Diabetes, you have too much sugar in your blood stream. So why is Twitch's blood sugar LOW? Well I'll tell you. This is where you need to listen carefully.

The owner said that he thought Twitch was doing ok a few days ago, but she started to vomit.

On a side note—apparently you humans think that vomiting is something that we do, like it's just a "cat thing" and it is ok. Well I have to tell you that it is NOT! Vomiting is not glamorous, and we cats are all about glamour! Did you ever notice the big production we make out of it, the horrible sounds, the twisted facial expressions? The whole body contractions? No! No self-respected feline would do that "just" because. It is "so NOT what we do!"

Anyway, poor Twitch, was vomiting—eating a little and still getting her insulin shots every day. She stopped wanting to eat and started to become a little "wobbly." So what does Mr. Owner decide to do to help her? He gives her MORE insulin thinking that was going to help ... But in the real world—that was making everything worse.

Here's the Raw Truth Recap of what happened ... Not eating > No outside source of glucose (sugar) > Give insulin > Whatever glucose is in the body gets lower > Still not eating > Give more insulin > Blood glucose gets even lower, cat gets weak, becomes wobbly > Still not eating > Give more insulin > Cat falls over and starts to twitch. Are you starting to see a pattern here?

So there you have it. Poor Twitch was being overdosed with her insulin and stayed in the hospital for almost a week. The good news is she slowly got better; it was touch and go for a little while. It ended up that she had a condition they call Pancreatitis. That is also a complicated process and apparently that is the place in the body where insulin in made. Simply stated, pancreatitis means inflammation of the pancreas. This caused her to vomit and have a lack of desire to eat.

After a few days of treatment, she started to look better and was almost back to her old self. She started to eat and groom herself as if nothing ever happened. She definitely used up a few of her lives. She was happily purring as she was placed in her travel box and she went home. So long Twitch.

Well, to help prevent this from happening again, Twitch was placed on a new type of diet and Mr. Owner got an education. He was very happy to have her back in his life and seemed grateful for the education that he received.

Oh, and in addition to that, here is some covert advice; mind you, I don't care much about this, but coming into the ER is not "free." There is an exchange of what they call *money for service*. I hear that being in the hospital can get costly. So, I guess keep that in mind.

Moral of the Story:

Knowledge always comes at a price. An ounce of prevention is definitely worth a pound of cure. A spoonful of sugar IS necessary for the medicine to go down (that's from Mary Poppins). AND ... last but not least ... more is not always better!

CHEECH

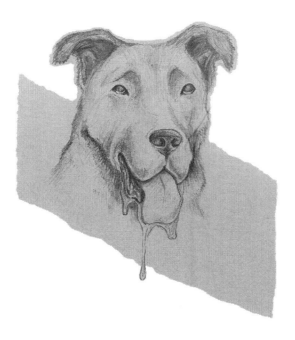

It was about 11 p.m. on a Friday night. I couldn't help but laugh when this dog came stumbling back into the treatment area. I don't know what kind of dog he was. He was all mixed up. He kind of looked like a small Labrador, mixed with German Shepard and a splash of Terrier thrown in. He was funny, bumping into things, dribbling pee everywhere, and every once in a while he would flinch like he saw something coming at him.

If I didn't know better, I would think he was hallucinating. Come to think of it, he probably was.

The doctor saw him and right away suspected foul play. She said he looked like he got into some THC, or Marijuana. Apparently where we live, it is legal for humans and used for medicinal purposes. This dude ate way too much. It must be the Lab in him! "Yo –Cheech," I said to him. "What's gotten into you?"

He looked at me like he was seeing lots of me and said he ate a plate of cookies and that they tasted great, but a little while afterward, he started to feel really weird.

"Yeah," I remarked. "You don't look so good, and besides, you're peeing all over yourself."

He then told me that he was cold and needed to go lie down somewhere really quiet and dark.

Well, as it turns out the "Great Doctorae" knew just what to do. They admitted him to the hospital, and they said they were worried about his heart rate and body temperature being so low and wanted to support and monitor him overnight. It turns out that Cheech had a double whammy. Not only was the marijuana not good for him, but the chocolate in the cookies could make him sick too. Poor Cheech.

The owner said it was his friend that brought over the cookies and he was mad—probably because he didn't get to eat any.

So good 'ol Cheech got his IV catheter, his fluids, a very soft bed, a heating blanket, and some other stuff. By the morning he was almost good as new. He wasn't his normal perky self, but at least he could walk a straight line and was able to go out to go to the bathroom. He ate a good breakfast and then went home.

Moral of the Story:

The Cookie Monster is not just a big blue fluffy thing. Keep all mind alerting, recreational treats placed in a secret vault under lock down. And, as "Man's Best Friend," what kind of friend wouldn't save you one cookie? Dogs—go figure!

SPEAKING OF DRUGS

Sometimes the hospital gets phone calls with random questions that the doctor answers. Here's one that will make you reconsider whether or not you want to be associated with the human species. This guy calls up and says, "I took some Ecstasy and my dog is licking my sweat. Is he going to want to have sex with me?" No joke. This is a true story! (For those of you who are unfamiliar with Ecstasy, it is a "recreation" drug—also called the "love pill.") The doctor glanced out into the room with a look of "Oh my god, did he just ask me that?" She responded with a straight face and deliberate tone. "Well Sir, if he does, just say NO."

Brilliant! Way to go Doc.

Ok as you all probably know, animals like to eat things. It is just who we are. We experience life through our noses and mouths. Sometimes it doesn't matter what we put into it. However, we cats tend to be much more selective.

Here's a Christmas story that I think you will enjoy.

A TREE, A CAT, A DOG, AND A BOX OF CHOCOLATE

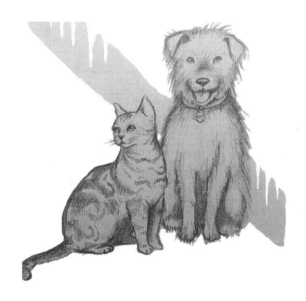

Sparkles (the cat) and Godiva (the dog) lived together. They were both brought in after the "Ruckus." What ruckus you ask? You know what they say. "When the cat's away the mice will play." I am not sure who said that or if it is even true, but I can tell you, when the owners are away the cat and dog will play!

Now this was back in the day when humans decorated their tress with tinsel. I think it was banned because of Sparkles, but chocolate is still around despite its propensity for danger.

Sparkles was really pretty. She was a grey and silver American shorthair with really cool stripy circle patterns on her side, and Godiva was very cute. She looked kind of like a longer haired female version of that dog Tramp from the movie *Lady and the Tramp*.

They came back into the treatment area together. I have to admit, they looked a little "Gangster," if you know what I mean. Sparkles was in a fancy pink and grey carrier and Godiva was on a sparkly leash. As Godiva walked in, I heard her saying something about this place reminding her of another place she went to in Brooklyn. All and all they looked pretty good. I asked them why they were here and Godiva said, "We got busted; now I guess we have to go to jail."

"What are YOU in for?" Sparkles asked me.

"That's a story for a different time," I said. "What did you guys do?"

"Well," hesitated Godiva, "here's how it all went down."

"You see, it was all Sparkles fault."

"Sure blame it on the cat," I thought.

"We were playing tag and Sparkles ran up the tree, I might have run into it as well while chasing her and the tree sort of ... well ... fell over. There was a mess—so Sparkles started to eat the tinsel. I thought, good idea let's clean this mess up! It was then that I noticed the big box of chocolate on the floor. The tree must have knocked it off the table on the way down. So like any good citizen, I started to help clean it up. It was all very innocent.

I cleaned up all the chocolate and Sparkles started eating tinsel like it was Sunday dinner at the Sopranos house! Just then the "cops" showed up. They were not happy! Frank, our guy human, had a scary look on his face. Guilty until proven innocent I suppose. But the lady human Linda, ran over to us and asked if we were ok. They argued and put us in the car. We drove for a little while, and here we are! Not exactly sure why."

"Well," I exclaimed, "buckle up. The ride's not over."

Just then the doctor came over. She examined them both and thought they both looked good, despite the obvious infraction.

The doctor left to go speak with Frank and Linda. After she got the story, she explained to them that she was going to "induce vomiting" to get the stuff out of their stomachs. She explained to them that chocolate is toxic to dogs and could be lethal, especially with the amount that Godiva ate, and the Tinsel needs to come out because it is not digestible and will get caught up in Sparkles intestines, which would result in her needing surgery.

The doctor warned them that sometimes cats don't vomit, and that they may have to get the tinsel out of her stomach some other way. Unfortunately, she may end up needing surgery. Needless to say Frank and Linda were far from happy, but they knew what they had to do.

The doctor gave Godiva an injection to make her vomit and within minutes her face became long, her ears drooped, and she started to drool. She looked really nauseous. Then all of a sudden she started to vomit. Oh my goodness! You should have seen the amount of chocolate that came up. It was like a river, and it smelled just like a Hershey's Kiss factory, (or should I say Godiva); there were even a few pieces of tinsel in there as well. "Good job, Godiva!" Everybody cheered as if they were so proud of her.

Next was Sparkles. The doctor gave her an injection and they waited for the big moment. Sparkles just sat there as if nothing was happening. (See, what did I tell you about cats and vomiting?). They waited a little while longer and after much discussion, the doctor told Frank and Linda that Sparkles didn't vomit and she would need to have a procedure they called Endoscopy. This is when they place a long tube like camera thing down into your stomach to look around and pull things out. Sorry Sparkles.

Like her name, she took the whole thing like a superstar. In the end, it all worked out. The chocolate was in the garbage where it belonged, and the ER team removed a big wadded up ball of tinsel from Sparkles stomach.

They gave it to Frank and Linda. I think they wanted to make an ornament out it for prosperity.

> ### *Moral of the Story:*
>
> *Before you leave mischief-makers home alone, especially during the holidays, secure the tree, nix the tinsel, and stash the chocolate. And when you go out shopping for ornaments, remember there are better places to get them that DON'T involve a cat's stomach.*

Since we are on the topic of eating things ...

D.A.

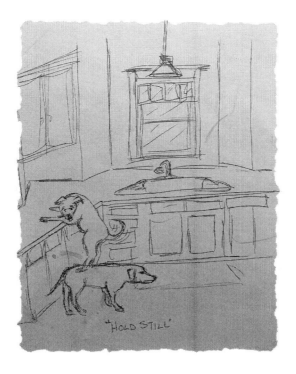

"HOLD STILL"

This is a story of great ingenuity and resourcefulness, and a little stupidity thrown in. There is a small twist, however. You see, this time it was the human that was the clever one. Remember I told you that the owners fill out information that goes on a sticker for the record?

Well not only did this male human write some funny stuff, he also drew a really great picture describing the incident. This is too good not to share.

Ok, so in comes this yellow Labrador Retriever, waging her tail, looking around happy, and smiling as if nothing happened. She thought she was just here to say hello. This is how her owner filled out the information:

Name: D.A.
Breed: Familiarus Canis
Mixed Breed: No
Sex: Female
Color: Blond (Go figure)
Date of Birth: Spawned Aug 03
Any known allergies: None – In Fact, she will eat anything.
Describe your pets diet: Anything, and I mean anything.
How long have you had your pet: Since she was hatched.
Describe your pets problems that brought you in here today: Terminally Stupid O.D.

The doctor asked him what "D.A." stood for he said "Dumb Ass," and the O.D. stood for over dose. As you can see from the picture, Miss D.A. coerced her canine compadre to stand there like a step stool so that she could climb on his back and get access to the counter. At that point, she got into the bottle of her compadre's heart medication and ate all the pills. It was just recently refilled so there were a lot in there. Yum! Classic Lab maneuver—doing a cool thing for a dumb reason.

It looked like Miss D.A. was potentially in a lot of trouble. Now, wait, hold up for a moment, let's take a step back and take a good look at this case.

I think we need to talk about this "Canine Companion" of hers. What were HIS motives? Was he just being helpful? Was it a blackmail situation? A bribe? Or was he just super smart, didn't like her, and wanted to see her off herself with his medication? Or perhaps he wanted to off himself and he needed her help in getting the medications, and she got carried away in the moment and ate them all! Your guess is as good as mine. Some things we never really get to know the answers to.

So, Miss D.A. got a chance to vomit up the medication. Unfortunately, not much came up, so she had to stay in the hospital and be treated and monitored for any ill effects of the prescription medication she enjoyed eating. She spent the next day in the hospital smiling and wagging her tail ... still, as if nothing ever happened. She went home to live another day.

Moral of the Story:

If you are planning on ingesting a lethal dose of prescription medication, always have a good support team to help execute your mission and a great doctor to save your Dumb Ass. And if you have a D.A. for a pet, it is always better to maintain a great sense of humor. .

LILLY

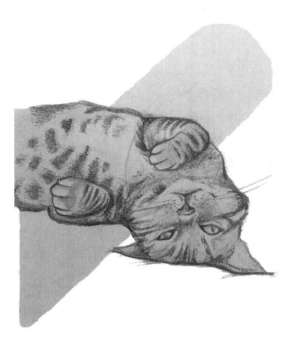

This one is a classic—and by this, I mean it typically happens. This Bengal cat comes in. I don't know if you have ever seen one, but she was special. She was brown, orange, tan, and black and bigger than most cats. She looked like the offspring of a mix of a mini tiger, a leopard, and an ocelot. I myself am quite awesome, and even I had cat envy. As she whooshed by she smelled like cat nip and flowers.

"Uh oh," said the good doctor as she examined her and noticed this fine yellow powder on her muzzle. Lilly looked ok for now, but the doctor asked to speak to the owners right away.

As it turns out, Lilly loved on some fresh flower lilies at home and the owners saw her eating some petals. The lady owner rushed her in because "Dr. Google" said that lilies were not good for kitties. It was good that she brought her cat in because they are indeed toxic. They can cause kitty kidney's to get really sick. They call it Renal failure in medical lingo. It is very serious. I have seen some cats get so sick that they needed dialysis! This cat definitely needed to stay in the hospital and get treatment.

The lady owner was very upset. What made things worse is that it was her one year anniversary with her new boyfriend and he brought her home this beautiful bouquet of flowers that had lilies in them. Poor guy. He was just trying to do something nice for his lady friend and here he goes poisoning her magnificent cat.

So she yelled at him, they argued, she cried ... and in the end Miss Lilly was admitted to the hospital for the care she needed. I feel Mr. Boyfriend paid for this in more ways than one. Good news is, about three days later, Miss Lilly went home. I have to admit, I did enjoy her being here. I'll miss our conversations ... and the way she smelled like Cat Nip.

Moral of the Story:

If you want to give your betrothed some flowers and she has a cat … buy fake ones. They last longer and don't try to kill you. Or just stick to the classic roses. We may like the smell, but the thorns are pokey, and as beautiful as they are, they are not likely to create a "feline fatale," or a "fatal feline."

Ok, back to the dogs. This is an even more romantic story.

ROCKY

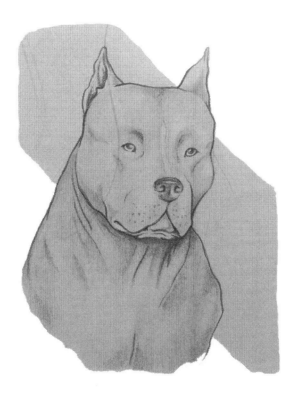

Meet Rocky. Rocky is a strong, muscular Pit Bull. He came swaging into the back area, showing off his muscles. I said to him, "Hey handsome, what brings you in here?"

Well I should have known better than to talk to him, because as soon as he got a whiff of me, I could see that he didn't want to be friends and was thinking about having a quick snack. All I'll say is that it was a good thing I was behind bars! Apparently, Rocky was a "people person" and didn't much like other dogs or cats. He got busy charming the nurses and the doctors with his fiendishly good looks.

So why was he here, looking so good? Well, it was a big night in the "Rocky" household. You see, him and his lady owner have been together for a long time. He really, really likes her. As it seems, she has this boyfriend who apparently wanted to be more than that. Humans have this ceremonial tradition where the male gives an offering to the female when he wants to marry her. I figure that it is kind of like some of us animals "mating for life." Anyway, Mr. Human, (I guess trying to be creative), placed this shiny ring on top of a cupcake. While he was paying attention to his love, Rocky saw an opportunity and ATE THE CUPCAKE!

Now I ask you ... was it the cupcake that Rocky wanted or was it the ring he didn't want his lady human to have? I don't know—I have to admit dogs can be pretty smart sometimes. So here he was, ring and all, and the guy wanted his ring back! So the good doctors decided that they would try to make Rocky vomit. They gave him an injection that made him really nauseous. Soon Rocky started to breath heavy and froth at the mouth. He had a sad look on his face. I didn't feel bad for him, being that he tried to eat ME not long before. The nurses placed a bunch of newspaper under him to catch the stuff. Within a few minutes, he started to vomit—and YUCK! Up came a bunch of dog food, what looked like a chewed up cupcake (paper and all), and ... no ring to be seen!

He was about to eat up his vomit when the nurses scooped it away from him. They placed the large mound of stuff on the table, put on some gloves, and started sifting through Rocky's vomit. That's what I call dedication. It seemed to take a while when one of them yelled out, "I found it!" Everybody cheered!

The diligent nurse washed the ring off in the sink and the doctor gave it back to the guy. It wouldn't be proper to give it to the lady owner just yet. That was his job. The guy was very grateful and they all went home. I don't know if Rocky was too happy. But I think his lady owner had a "heart to heart" conversation with him.

Moral of the Story:

If you want to propose, consider having a private moment. And when Beyoncé said, "If you like then you should have put a ring on it," I think she meant a finger and not a cupcake.

_*~*~*_

GETTING SOME PURRSPECTIVE

Although it may not be obvious due to our external nonchalant *cattitude*, there are some moments in time that make one take a step back and get some perspective about life. Sometimes, when I am feeling sorry for myself, contemplating all the "woe is me" moments, I think about this next story. It is about a very brave canine soul who came in because of a stupid thing some other human did.

NERO

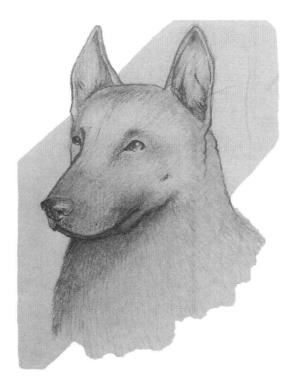

Nero is a Belgian Melanios. He is not just any dog; he is a Working Dog. Yes you heard me, he has a job to do and he takes it very seriously. He is a Police Dog—a K-9 Cop. What makes him so special? Besides his good looks, his unique athleticism, extraordinary skill level, and historically keen intelligence ... Well, all I can say is when I first met him, I questioned my own purpose and found myself in a mini-existential crisis.

"Two techs to the front STAT!" cried the overhead page.

He didn't come in proud; he came in on the gurney. He was injured in the line of duty. He was in very bad shape. You see, these dogs go through very special and rigorous training. Nero was part of the K-9 Criminal Apprehension Unit.

As he passed by me on the gurney, he was conscious but lying there very still and breathing very heavy; there was blood all over his face. He seemed to look at me, but I don't think he really saw me. Word had it that Nero was shot. Within moments there were a swarm of doctors and nurses around him that began to stabilize him in the magical way that they do. Placing IV catheters, giving fluids, administering pain medications, and taking blood to check his values. They also hooked him up to this machine called an ECG, otherwise known as an Electrocardiogram. It shows the electrical heartbeat and rhythm—it makes a sort of musical beeping sound that is comforting when all is well.

His beeping was very fast. The amazing doctor said he was in shock and while Nero was being stabilized, she was trying to find the source of the blood on his face. It appeared to keep bleeding. As the cleaning progressed, she found wounds on his muzzle, by his nose, and in the inside of his mouth that went to the side of his face just underneath his eye. There was a lot of bleeding, and they found an artery that might have been the culprit. They said they needed to try to "ligate it," which means tie a string around it, or as they like to call it, a suture. The doctors and nurses were focused and on task. They tried, but they could not get to the artery without surgery. It was too deep inside the wound.

Nero was very cooperative, probably from the shock of the trauma and the sedative pain medications he received, or maybe because he was really smart and knew that they were trying to help him. Anyway, the doctor packed off the wound, instructed the nurse to apply pressure, and when Nero seemed more stable, she spoke to the officer that brought him in.

Now to give a little back history, these dogs are trained to be with and work with one specific human. The officer that brought him in was that guy. The officer explained to the doctor that they were involved in a shooting and another officer was also shot during the attempted arrest. Unfortunately, he was at the human ER. We weren't able to get the whole story, *why* they were there, *if* they apprehended the assailant (that means "got the bad guy" in police talk). That information was considered "police business," and he said he wasn't allowed to talk about it. The officer did however want the bullet retrieved from Nero, if they found it, for a ballistic analysis report.

The doctor explained that Nero would need surgery after he was stabilized to explore the gunshot area, repair whatever damage they could, and hopefully retrieve the bullet. They took an X-ray of his head before surgery and found out that he also had some fractures to his nose and facial bones, and that there were many fragments of metal but no actual bullet.

They took him to surgery that day and the surgeon did what she could to repair the trauma. He did well during the procedure; the fractures in his face would heal over time. Nero was heavily sedated on pain medications for a couple of days post operatively, or post-op as we say here in the ER. After a couple more days, he recovered, was able to eat soft foods, and was scheduled to go home. The sad thing is that his human co-worker wasn't as fortunate as he was and didn't make it out of the ER. He died in the line of duty.

Nero recovered fully but lost the sight from his left eye, secondary to the trauma. He earned a medal of honor and was able to retire from active duty, but he was very sad. From the look on his face, you can tell that he felt alone and somewhat responsible. He lost a good comrade; they all did.

I felt really bad for him and tried to cheer him up. I told him that he was the bravest dog I have ever met, and he was considered a hero, amongst humans and animals alike. I also told him that they caught the bad guy that shot them both. (We found that out a few days after he was here in the hospital). He put on a brave face, gave me a nod, and left with his partner officer that brought him in.

Nero went on to live with this officer. He had a nice home, a big yard, and a great big bed to relax in. He was a really nice human.

Moral of the Story:

Sometimes you find yourself in the wrong place at the right time, or the right place at the wrong time, or the right place at the right time, or even the wrong place at the wrong time. Regardless ... It is good to be grateful for and remember all the brave people and animals out there that every day put their own lives on the line to save others, because not everybody is as lucky as us cats to have nine lives.

_*~*~*_

NOT SO "BEACHY" AFTER ALL

Ok, well, we all know dogs love going to the beach. There are so many things to do there—playing Frisbee, catching balls, surfing. Yes, dogs can Hang 16. (They technically have thumbs, but they are pretty useless and often, just get in the way). I heard that Huntington Beach in Southern California hosts an annual surf competition. I have even heard that there are Bulldogs who enter. May wonders never cease to amaze! Well, everything is fun and games—until it is not.

Let me tell you about Scuba.

SCUBA

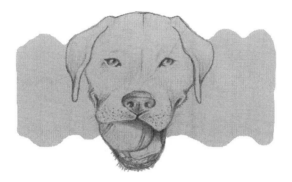

In comes Scuba on the gurney. He was wet and covered in sand. Ok, you guessed it; he just came from the beach. Scuba was a Golden Retriever who lived for the beach and for chasing balls. Now sometimes those two things don't always mix well. He was having trouble breathing and his tongue was on the blueish side. Not good! The doctors rushed over to examine him.

The team got busy doing all sorts of things. One was giving him oxygen, another was drying him up and trying to get the sand off, and others were placing the IV catheter and getting blood work. Yep, these guys were pros.

The doctor went in to talk to the owner, who, by the way, was also wet and covered with sand and apparently believed that shoes were optional. As it turns out, Scuba and friend were playing fetch in the ocean for a while.

Now, you have to understand that some dogs have a pathologic attachment to balls and will not stop until they drop. Scuba was one of those dogs. He got himself so carried away that he ended up inhaling and swallowing a bunch of ocean. He was probably trying to get in touch with his inner fish. The doctors call this a near drowning.

Scuba vomited up large amounts of salt water and in the process inhaled some of it as well. They call this "Aspiration." Apparently when you inhale stuff from your stomach you can get an infection in your lungs called Pneumonia.

Scuba had salt water in his lungs, developed pneumonia, and let's not forget to mention what proceeded to be evacuated from the other end. Trust me; you don't want to go there. Poor Scuba. He did not look like he was feeling well. He was hospitalized and stayed in the oxygen tank for four days. He slowly recovered and was discharged a few days later.

He was very happy when he was able to go home. He left wagging his tail and carrying his ball. Yes, the ball stayed with him in the hospital for moral support.

Being that Southern California is considered a beachy place there are many dogs that come into the hospital for beach related incidents. He was one of the lucky ones. Some of these dogs need to go on ventilators, and some never make it. At least his name wasn't Lucky ... that's never a good sign.

Moral of this Story:

Even though your dog loves to play, be aware of their limits, because they rarely pay attention to that. They find inspiration from the Eveready Bunny. And just because your dog likes to swim, don't confuse them with a gill bearing aquatic creature.

SUPERMAN

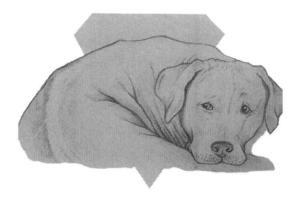

This is a sad but touching story. This sort of things happens way too often, and although I am partial to cats, I do feel bad for the brave canines that come in here.

There is a big machine out there in the world; it is called a pickup truck. It moves around when humans get in, and they like to put lots of stuff in the open back, including their dogs. Now most of the time these are big, strong looking dogs. It is rare, and probably unheard of, to see a Toy Poodle or a Maltese hanging around in the back. So here is how I met Superman. The overhead page announced, "Two techs to the front STAT!" Next thing I saw was this dog being rolled in.

He was flat out on the gurney. He was lying there panting, and he was covered in blood, dirt, and grease. It was hard to see where the blood was coming from. It was even hard to tell what kind of dog he was. He sort of looked like a Labrador mixed with a Rhodesian Ridgeback because he had a cool little mohawk down along the top of his back.

The elite team of doctors and nurses were all over him, and everyone was doing something different. I heard one of the doctors say that he was in shock and called up front for an approval for a "critical." That is a quick way to get permission legally and financially to treat the patient. It also lets the owner know right away just how serious things are.

The doctors and nurses where very busy placing catheters, giving him oxygen, taking blood for lab tests, cleaning wounds, and giving fluids and medications. Oh those wonderful pain medications! After they cleaned him up a bit, they found out where all the blood came from. He had a very large wound under his armpit, his paws were bleeding, and he bit his tongue. They spent the next 10-15 minutes getting him out of shock and stabilizing him.

Even though he was heavily sedated, they said that he was stabilizing but still considered critical. The doctor left to go talk to the owner (who we will call Dave), while Superman was in Radiology getting X-rays taken.

The doctor came back with a very serious look on her face. She checked on Superman, looked at the radiographs, and then went back in the room to speak with Dave. It seemed like she was in there for a really long time.

You see, poor Superman was riding in the back of this pickup truck and had a long leash around his neck that was tied up to one part of the truck. I don't know how fast they were going, but Superman decided that he wanted to fly. He must have seen something really interesting ... like a squirrel or a stick. Anyway, he jumped off of the truck. The leash got caught around his front leg. He was trying to run alongside the moving truck, all the while being tangled in the leash. Dave finally realized what was happening, stopped the truck, got Superman back into the truck, and rushed him into the ER.

Can you say OUCH! Good thing he got his arm stuck because he would have hung himself if he didn't. There is ALWAYS a bright side, it COULD have been worse! So as it turns out he had a broken shoulder, a large gaping wound under his arm, and some other bumps and bruises.

The doctor told Dave that he was going to need intensive care and multiple surgeries and he would need to be in the hospital for at least a week, possibly longer. After their conversation, the doctor brought him back to see his dog friend on the treatment table.

When Dave went over to Superman he raised his head, tried to lick his face, and even wagged his tail a little. Dave, filled with sadness, tears, and guilt gave Superman a big kiss, told him that he was very sorry this happened and would do whatever was needed to help get him well, and reminded him to keep strong.

Superman was strong and a trooper. He always maintained a really great attitude. As the days went by, he was less and less critical. He got his surgeries, and Dave made sure to visit him every day, reminding him of how much he loved him and was wishing him well. He would tell him stories about future experiences they were going to have together. We all liked Dave and Superman very much.

It took about eight days and although Superman was ready to go home, he still had some healing to do. Dave was going to take him to get physical rehabilitation and cool things like Acupuncture, and Cold LASER therapy. He even got to sit in the front seat from now on.

Superman got lots of kisses and hugs before he left. I even gave him a high six. Oh, did I mention I have six toes on each of my front paws? That's right. They call me a Polydactyl, but more about me later.

> ### So the Moral of this Story:
>
> *If your dog rides in the back of a pickup truck then look into getting a really good safety harness or restraint system. "Dr. Google" can help you with that. Also, it pays to look into getting Health Insurance. Dave had some, and it really helped him out a lot. AND ... Remember—even though some dogs are named after superheroes, DOGS CAN'T FLY!*

Here's a funny story about an animal that could fly but couldn't.

SUZIE

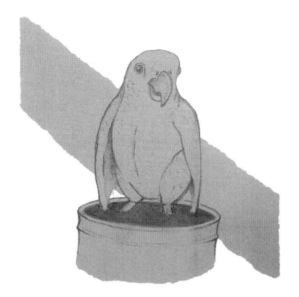

Suzie was a very beautiful Amazon parrot. She was mostly green, but her head was yellow with some blue by her nose, which is called a beak. She came in looking like a statue. No really. She was a statue, stuck in a block of stuff not moving. Want to hear that story?

Well, Suzie was home with her owner flying around, and her owner was in the bathroom, preparing to wax the hair from her body. Apparently this is a certain ritual that female humans go through.

Anyway, Suzie flies into the bathroom and lands on, or in, the block of melted wax ... ouch! AND proceeded to get STUCK! Her feet and the tip of her wings were in the wax. The owner panicked and grabbed Suzie in the wax box, ran out of the house, placed her in the basket of her bicycle, and proceeded to head to the ER.

It took her a little while to get to the hospital and by that time, Suzie was very statuesque! She seemed pretty calm for a bird stuck in a block of wax. I think she knew that freedom was in her future.

SO ... the good doctors deliberated for a short while to decide on the best way to get her out. They proceeded to chip away at the block, and as they got closer to Suzie's feet and wings, they took out some special liquid that helped dissolve the wax. They were so meticulous during that part. It looked like Michelangelo carving the David.

Suzie was amazing! She was calm and cooperative the whole time. It took a little over four hours to get her free and remove all the wax off her feet and feathers. Afterwards, she was happy and flapping all over. She was good as new. I'm not sure how she got home in her bicycle, being that she was free to fly around, but apparently they made it home safely.

> **Moral of the Story:**
>
> **If you want a "Brazilian," consider taking a trip to South America that doesn't involve a bird and a block of wax.**

Birds may be built for flying but we cats have been known to try.

FLYING CATS

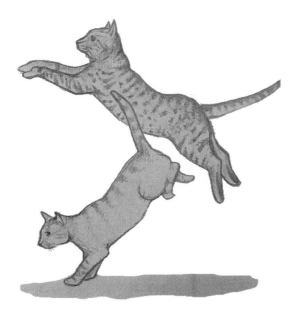

I have seen cats fly. There is a saying that cats will always land on their feet. Now, that is not exactly true; it depends upon a few variables, one of them being what we might hit on the way down. But seriously, it is all about the aerodynamics. Allow me to introduce Crash and Eddie. They were two very typical looking Tabbies.

Take Crash—he lived on the fifth floor of a ten-story building. He had a balcony that the owner said he would sit out on and sunbathe. I don't think that she thought that one day he would ... jump! Well, Crash spent some time watching birds, and one day he tried to grab one. He thought he could fly!

Well, as it turned out he fell, five stories down. Lucky for him he didn't hit anything on the way, except the grassy ground. He did land feet side down but also suffered some pretty bad injuries. He wounded his chin, split his hard palate (that is the roof of your mouth), and got what is called a "Pneumothorax." That is a big medical word for having air in your chest cavity that is NOT inside your lungs. When the air is trapped in that space, it is hard to breathe because it creates pressure on the lungs and they cannot inflate. Not a good situation.

The good doctor gave him some of that pain medication, removed the air from his chest cavity with a needle and syringe, cleaned up his wounds, and placed him inside the Oxygen tank. He looked pretty good. They said the inside of his mouth will heal on its own. They kept him in the hospital for a couple of days, and then he went home.

Then there was Eddie. Eddie lived downtown in an apartment in a really tall building. He lived on the nineteenth floor. He too had a balcony. He wasn't allowed on it. One day there was a small opening in the door and he wiggled through it. And, well, you guessed it; he jumped, or fell (the story is not clear, but I am sure there was a bird involved).

SO, what happened to Eddie? He too, like Crash, had a free falling experience and didn't hit anything until he hit the ground. SMASH! But wait! You can take a breath and open your eyes. NOTHING happened to Eddie! Well almost nothing. Not a scratch, bruise, or bump. He did, however, break his upper canine tooth. Can you believe it? I didn't think so.

Allow me to explain. You see, we cats can "land on our feet" because we have the ability to execute a maneuver called a "righting reflex" in space. There are some really cool slow–mo videos out there if you want to see it. Now, if we are falling from a short distance, we are hitting the ground upon acceleration bracing for impact. And, well, we end up hurting ourselves. Now, if we fall from higher up, say more than six stories, we not only "right" ourselves but get the chance to achieve what they call "terminal velocity" and "free fall," sort of like a flying squirrel, and hit the ground not only at a slower speed (due to the increase in the drag factor), but also in a more relaxed state. Hence sustaining much less severe injuries. How's that for an explanation!

Even though Eddie looked good, the doctors wanted to keep him for observation overnight. I heard he ended up seeing a Veterinary Dentist and getting a gold cap on his broken tooth.

Note, that even though the concepts of aerodynamics are true, not all cats are as fortunate as Eddie.

There are a few variables involved and the degree of trauma depends upon what they may hit or get caught on, on the way down, how high they started, and of course landing tactics, and potential preexisting injuries.

Keep in mind that this DOES NOT apply to dogs. They always go SPLAT!

Moral of the Story:

Even though cats have an amazing ability to become aerodynamic, it is NEVER a good idea to throw your cat off the balcony to see if it can fly. Also, if one should jump, don't assume the worst and PLEASE go and check to see what happened. Always seek professional, medical help before deciding if your "stuntman dare devil" should quit his job of being a cat.

_*~*~*_

Speaking of dogs and balconies, let me tell you about Spidey.

SPIDEY

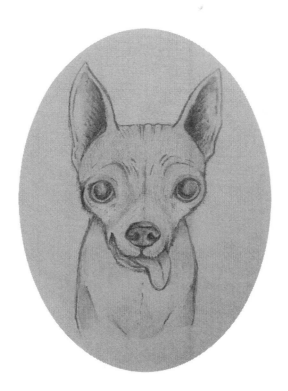

Spidey was a 17-year-old Chihuahua! That's OLD. Did you know that there is an ACTUAL place in Mexico called Chihuahua that all these little guys came from? Anyway, Spidey was small, skinny, and blind. He had a thing called cataracts. He didn't do too much.

Most days he spent sleeping, eating, and occasionally walking, or creaking, over to his inside grass area to go to the bathroom. Have you heard of that? It is like a litter box for dogs but more like an inside park. You humans can be so creative at times.

Spidey lived on the second story of an apartment complex. One sunny day in October, Spidey decided he would take a walk onto the balcony, something he would never usually do. Maybe he wanted to get some fresh air, maybe he wanted to feel the sun upon his little old body, or perhaps he was thinking about a grand finale. It is really hard to say exactly what he was thinking about, but that day Spidey decided to walk off the balcony.

As you can imagine, it didn't end well for old Spidey. He did, however, survive the fall, but he was pretty broken up and not very alert. The good doctor immediately examined him, gave him some pain medication as soon as he came to the back, and then went to go speak with his owners. The doctor spent a while consulting with Spidey's people and in the end they decided it was best to help him on his journey towards his new life, over that proverbial Rainbow Bridge.

You see, veterinarians are allowed to perform a thing they call Euthanasia. It is a way for animals to have a peaceful and dignified passing into the next "realm" of life, if you will. We cats are very familiar with it. You may notice us staring off into the distance at times. That is us mediating and doing cool things like time-space travel. We can get into that another time.

Well, Spidey had a very peaceful transition in the arms of those who loved him. It was all very touching ... really. I think Spidey ended up getting what he ultimately wanted. Rest in Peace Spidey.

> ### *Moral of this Story:*
>
> *Never underestimate the will power of the seemingly frail. And there are things in life that we may never fully understand, but if you look into your hearts, you will find the answers.*

—*~*~*—

That is the Zen side of me. SO, there you have it. That was the last one ... for now. Don't worry ... there are always plenty more *Stupid Things you Humans Do* to talk about.

MY PERSONAL STORY

What? You want to know what happened to me. Well ... Since you asked so nicely. After my four-month quarantine was up, I entered The Blood Donorship Special Ops Program. I got moved to the cool cat tree area with the great view. I met some of my fellow squad-mates. They were really cool cats! We shared our stories and bonded over our own personal tragedies.

This dude named Crush became my best bud. He is orange like me. He has this wonky back leg that doesn't work right. He says it doesn't hurt; it's just not as good as it used to be. He has trouble scratching the side of his face. I help him out with that most of the time; other times I like to watch him try to do it. Hey—what are friends for if you can't offer them a little encouragement now and then?

He said he got his name after his pelvis got crushed when a garage door slammed down on top of him (yep, just another stupid human thing to do). He too had surgery, and even though he's not sporting a Pagina like me, he has a cool metal plate holding his pelvis together. His pelvis never healed quite right, hence the wonky leg.

He's donated his blood a bunch of times. He said it wasn't so bad. The doctors give you an injection that makes you really sleepy, and then afterwards when they are done, you get to eat some extra yummy food.

Hmm ... I wasn't too excited about this whole thing, but I was ok with the idea of community service. During my quarantine, I certainly got a chance to see all the situations of cats that would need to use some of my wonder-blood.

Shortly after I started the program, I was called for duty. There was a feline in distress that needed my help. Oh, in case you didn't know, cats have three blood types; A, B and AB, (which is very rare). I'm an A. I guess it stands for Awesome! Anyway, they were going to take some blood from me and gave me the stuff that makes you sleepy; they call it a sedative. This was given so that I would be absolutely still while they did what they had to do.

Well, the whole thing didn't get very far. Apparently, I wasn't as ok with this as I thought I'd be. After they gave me the sedative, I felt super weird and I sort of freaked out ... in a really major way, enough for them to seriously reconsider my services. They said I had a very unusual reaction to the medication and thought it best that I didn't participate. So as it turns out, I got released from the Special Ops Donorship Program. They called it an "Entry Level Separation"—no harm no foul, just didn't work out. I still feel loved.

I have to admit—even though I felt bad, I was kind of glad I was able to leave the hospital sooner than I thought. Now I was officially up for adoption. It didn't take long for somebody to want to take me home, me being such a Stud Muffin and all. Heck, they were even fighting over me.

In the end, I went home with one of the amazing, elite ER doctors; the one that I told you about in my stories. I always felt we had some kind of kinship going on. She always gave me extra attention and was in support of my secret likings for muffins. Yep. This was a match made in heaven.

I said farewell to my best bud Crush. I promised him that I would be there for him when he was ready for discharge. So I left the hospital with my new best human and she took me home.

Now, you may think that this is the start of a beautiful thing, and eventually it was, but let me recap my life for you. I started in the wild, ended up behind bars, and now was in a house. Don't get me wrong, I love my new home. It is just that there are things in there that I never knew about.

For a short while, I was in stealth survival mode as I got accustomed to the terrain. I squeezed myself into the smallest places I could find to obtain optimum observation and surveillance without being detected.

I did this from various places throughout the house for a couple of weeks.

In homes they have these large rectangle things—big, loud, and filled with images of unsuspecting threats. There are also these things that were above me that spin fast and blow air, not to mention this terribly loud machine that sucks stuff up and has a tail that looks like a snake. I have battled with that one a number of times.

Oh and I almost forgot ... in homes there are more humans! Small ones called CHILDREN. It was with one of them that I discovered my hidden talent and propensity for a thing called "Dress up."

Yes, it took me a little while to adjust to home life. But I got the hang of it. I now like to watch the cooking shows on the television, I sit under the fans on hot days, and I take naps in all the best places. I eat the best food and always look forward to "Sashimi Sundays." I get to hang out in a great back yard with the butterflies, and take surveillance in my favorite tree. I have since perfected my favorite past time ... you guessed it ... napping! Yep, my life is pretty good.

My humans are great, and I pretty much run the place, hence my nick name *King Queso*. They added the Meso McFuzzy Butt part ... I guess because...well, have you seen my butt? It is indeed fuzzy. I am however, an avid groomer and an expert in yoga.

When I am outside and it is time for dinner, my human calls for me, "King Queso Meso McFuzzy Butt, you get your fuzzy butt back home right now!" and, well, when I hear that ... I always come running.

Yep, life in the kingdom is pretty great. Not to mention that I also cohabitate with a bunch of other critters. There are a couple of geckos, a rat, some fish and...Oh, as for my best bud Crush? Well, he's busy right now napping in the sun room.

It wasn't long after I came to this fine establishment that he completed his active duty. He was really happy to see me again, and before you knew it, we were running around chasing each other, enjoying our daily wrestling matches. For the most part, I always win, except when he would sneak an attack with his wonky foot.

Oh man, he's the best! It's a good life.

Well, that is the end of my tale. Thanks for listening to my stories! I hope you enjoyed them and maybe learned a thing or two. Keep a lookout for my next book, *Cat's Don't Cough up Hairballs and Other Fun Facts.*

Until then ... Ciao Meow!

MY AWESOME HUMAN'S BIO

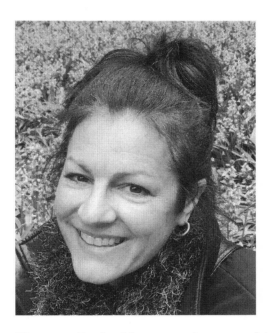

This is my Human. I asked her to write something about herself, but she said that she would be happy if I did it. As it turns out, she is quite unique. Her name is Barrie Sands. She grew up in Brooklyn, New York. She has been a veterinarian for over 25 years. After graduating from veterinary school, she completed an Internship in Small Animal Medicine and Surgery at the prestigious Animal Medical Center in Manhattan (That's NYC not Kansas).

She worked in private practice in New York City for four years and then moved to San Diego where she has been working for the last twenty years as one of the elite Emergency Critical Care doctors.

She is also trained in Traditional Chinese Medicine, is certified in Acupuncture, and has a successful holistic practice. She has been practicing holistic medicine for the last 14 years, utilizing things like medicinal botany, or Chinese herbology, nutrition, various physical rehabilitation modalities, and this thing they call Energy medicine. I'm pretty sure she learned that from cats. She is able to integrate the best of both worlds—the East and the West to allow for the greatest opportunities for healing.

I think after being a conventional doctor for so long and not seeing the wellness that she wanted, she decided to embrace all aspects of healing. Believe me, I have seen it. I am sure she would be happy for me to share some of her Eastern medicine stories. She says that working in the ER is the Yang and working in her holistic practice is the Yin ... whatever that means.

She is also a certified Coach from the Institute of HeartMath and teaches other humans techniques to be able to go into what they call Heart Brain Coherence. It has something to do with stress management.

Besides hanging around with me, she, or I should say (we), live with her husband, her two children (I do like them a lot), Crush, and those other critters I told you about (they are ok – they just don't do too much).

She is also a fantastic cook! She says it is one of her passions. I always keep her company when she prepares the meals—she likes to share! She loves to do yoga with me, and on occasion we get to take naps together. For me that's just purrfect!

In the future, we plan on collaborating on other books about Western and Eastern medicine, a cookbook and of course, amazing animal stories. I, for one, plan on being very busy.

* * *

Oh, and if you are wondering about the cool sketches throughout the book; they were created by one of the receptionists at the hospital. She was always really nice to me and she can draw. Her name is Annamarie Go. She's also going to school to be some sort of a radiologic technician (whatever that is). I told her she is wasting her talents and should consider going into illustration. Anyway, I'm glad she decided to draw for me. I really like her.

Thanks Annamarie!

* * *

I also want to honor the graphic designer. She is the one who helped create the cool graphics with the sketches. Her name is Joyous King and she also works at the hospital as the head nurse of the internal medicine department. I say she helped because I was trying to do something artistic. As you know we cats have a natural predisposition for the arts, especially when we push things off of counters and create an ingenious transformation of a vase into a mosaic. Graphic designing wasn't working out so well for me. Joy,(as she is referred to by her friends) being gifted and kind hearted, offered to help me and patiently explained that Photoshop was apparently not designed for cats, even ones with six toes.

Thanks Joy!

EPILOGUE

Dr. Barrie Sands

Here are some definitions, according to Webster's Dictionary:

Stupid: *having or showing a great lack of intelligence or common sense*

Stupidity: *a behavior that lacks a good sense, or judgment.*

Ignorance: *a lack of knowledge or information.*

Awareness: *knowledge or perception of a situation or fact.*

I do hope you enjoyed reading some of Señor Queso's stories. It was fun trying to choose through all the stories that he wanted to talk about.

On a more serious note, the emergency room is not a place where most people want to spend their time, emotions, and finances. When they do, the event can have profound effects in ways that may not be readily apparent. And like so many things in life that happen, mistakes and unfortunate events can be prevented with a little more knowledge, common sense, and awareness. That being said, please keep in mind, besides some of the stories you have read, animals present to the ER for a variety of other reasons; such as decompensation or exacerbation of chronic metabolic medical conditions. These cases were not the focus of this book.

There are however, situations and events that occur with our pets, because they are silly, carefree, and live in the moment with true abandonment; that sometimes—stuff just happens. It is important to take those moments in stride, try to maintain a sense of humor, work together to help each other through the tough times, learn from our mistakes, and most importantly, remember to forgive—ourselves and each other.

* * *

An Old Man said,

"Erasers are made for those who make mistakes."

A Youth said,

"Erasers are made for those who are willing to correct their mistakes."

And as Señor Queso says,

"Mistakes made are just opportunities to strive for purrfection, and if at all possible, blame it on the dog."

~ *The End* ~

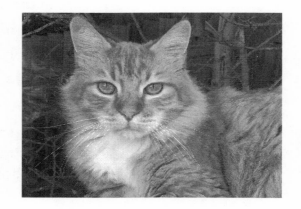

ACKNOWLEDGEMENTS

I want to thank Señor Queso for being a large and wonderful part of my life and for trusting me to write this book.

I want to thank the amazing group of doctors, veterinarian technicians, and support staff that work so hard every day to help make a difference in the lives of animals and their human companions.

I am thankful to my artistic team; Annamarie Go, and Joyous King, whose time and dedication was much appreciated.

I am grateful to the Self-Publishing School, and my mentor Scott Allan, my editor Sky Rodio Nuttall and formatter Debbie Lum for helping me get the book out into the world.

I am ever thankful for my family who has supported me throughout this process.

And last, I would like to give thanks for all the people that have come into the emergency room, for without them I would not have any stories to write.

Made in the USA
Monee, IL
03 December 2019